DR LINDA SMITH

HEALTH GUIDE ON HOW TO PREVENT AND MANAGE HEART DISEASE

Contents

I

Part One

1

INTRODUCTION

Understanding the Basic

Coronary illness, otherwise called cardiovascular sickness, is an expansive term that includes a scope of conditions influencing the heart and veins. It's a huge worldwide wellbeing concern and a main source of death in numerous nations. To successfully forestall and oversee coronary illness, understanding its principal aspects is fundamental.

1. The Cardiovascular System:

At the center of coronary illness lies the cardiovascular framework, a mind boggling network liable for shipping blood, oxygen, and supplements all through the body. The key parts include:

- **The Heart:** A strong organ that goes about as a siphon, impelling blood into flow.

- **Blood Vessels:** Supply routes, veins, and vessels structure a multifaceted parkway framework for blood stream.

- **Blood:** A crucial liquid conveying oxygen, supplements, chemicals, and byproducts.

2. Types of Heart Disease:

Coronary illness is certainly not a solitary condition yet a class including different problems. Normal sorts include:

- **Coronary Course Infection (CAD):** Portrayed by the restricting or blockage of coronary veins, which supply blood to the heart muscle.

- **Heart Failure:** When the heart can't siphon blood productively, prompting weakness and liquid development.

- **Arrhythmias:** Sporadic heart rhythms that might be excessively quick (tachycardia) or excessively sluggish (brady-cardia).

- **Valvular Heart Diseases:** Issues with heart valves, influencing blood stream all through the heart.

**3. Causes and Hazard Factors:

Coronary illness commonly results from a mix of variables, including:

- **Genetics:** A family background of coronary illness can expand your gamble.

- **Way of life Choices:** Smoking, an unfortunate eating regimen, absence of activity, unnecessary liquor utilization, and stress add to coronary illness.

- **Clinical Conditions:** Conditions like hypertension, ele-vated cholesterol, weight, and diabetes are huge gamble factors.

**4. Symptoms:

Side effects of coronary illness can shift broadly founded on the particular condition yet may include:

Chest Agony or Discomfort: Frequently alluded to as angina.

- **Brevity of Breath:** Particularly during actual work or very still.-

Fatigue: Feeling uncommonly drained, even with in-significant effort.

- **Unpredictable Heartbeat:** Palpitations or vibes of skipped thumps.

5. Counteraction and Management: Forestalling coronary illness and overseeing existing circumstances require a diverse methodology, including:

- **Solid Lifestyle:** Taking on a fair eating routine, participating in customary activity, and stopping smoking.

- **Medications:** Relying upon the condition, drugs like statins, blood thinners, or beta-blockers might be recommended.

- **Careful Interventions:** now and again, methods like angioplasty, stent position, or sidestep a medical procedure might be vital.

Understanding the fundamentals of coronary illness is the establishment for settling on informed decisions about your heart wellbeing. Ordinary clinical exams, risk factor evaluations, and way of life changes can go far in forestalling and overseeing coronary illness actually.

2

RISK ELEMENTS FOR CORONARY ILLNESS, RECOGNIZING YOUR VULNERABILITY

Coronary illness is much of the time impacted by a mix of hereditary, way of life, and natural variables. Distinguishing your particular gamble factors is an essential move toward forestalling and dealing with this condition really. In this conversation, we'll investigate the key gamble factors and how to perceive your weaknesses.

1. Family History:

One of the most grounded marks of coronary illness risk is your family ancestry. If direct relations, like guardians or kin, have had coronary illness, particularly early on, your gamble might be higher because of shared hereditary qualities and ecological impacts.

2. Age:

Age is a non-modifiable gamble factor. As you become older, the gamble of coronary illness normally increments. It's vital to be more careful about heart wellbeing as you age and consider normal check-ups and way of life changes.

3. Gender:

Men will quite often be at a higher gamble for coronary illness than pre-menopausal ladies. Notwithstanding, after menopause, ladies' gamble builds and can move toward that of men. Understanding these orientation related contrasts can assist with fitting preventive measures.

4. Hypertension (Hypertension):

Raised pulse overwhelms the heart and veins. Standard checking and the executives of hypertension are basic in lessening your gamble of coronary illness.

5. Elevated Cholesterol Levels:

Elevated degrees of LDL (low-thickness lipoprotein) cholesterol, frequently alluded to as "terrible" cholesterol, can prompt the development of plaque in your supply routes, expanding the gamble of coronary illness.

6. Smoking:

Smoking is a significant supporter of coronary illness. The synthetic compounds in tobacco can harm veins and diminish the oxygen-conveying limit of blood. Stopping smoking is one of the best ways of bringing down your gamble.

7. Diabetes:

Diabetes, especially type 2 diabetes, is firmly connected to coronary illness. Raised glucose levels can harm veins over the long haul. Appropriate diabetes the board is fundamental for heart wellbeing.

8. Heftiness and Overabundance Weight:

Conveying abundance weight, particularly around the midsection, expands the gamble of coronary illness. Keeping a sound load through diet and exercise can relieve this gamble.

9.** Poor Diet:**

An eating regimen high in soaked and trans fats, salt, and added sugars can add to coronary illness. Perceiving the significance of a heart-sound eating routine wealthy in natural products, vegetables, entire grains, and lean proteins is vital.

10. Actual Inactivity:

A stationary way of life is a gamble factor for coronary illness. Standard actual work fortifies the heart and works on by and large cardiovascular wellbeing.

11. Stress:

Constant pressure can unfavorably affect heart wellbeing. Figuring out how to oversee pressure through unwinding procedures, care, or guiding can be useful.

12. Unreasonable Liquor Consumption:

While moderate liquor utilization might have a few cardiovascular advantages, unreasonable drinking can expand the gamble of coronary illness. Understanding what comprises moderate drinking is critical.

By recognizing these put factors in your life in danger and working with your medical services supplier, you can make a customized plan to decrease your weaknesses to coronary illness. Standard wellbeing check-ups, way of life changes, and drug when fundamental are fundamental stages toward a heart-solid future

3

ROLE OF GENETICS IN HEART HEALTH

Hereditary qualities assumes a critical part in heart wellbeing. Here are a few central issues to consider:

1. **Genetic Predisposition**: A few people acquire qualities that increment their gamble of heart illnesses, like coronary course infection or arrhythmias. These hereditary elements can make an individual more helpless to heart-related conditions.

2. **Familial Patterns**: Heart wellbeing frequently runs in families. In the event that direct relations like guardians or kin have a background marked by coronary illness, your gamble might be higher because of shared hereditary variables and way of life propensities.

3. **Genetic Mutations**: Certain hereditary changes can straightforwardly affect heart wellbeing. For example, transformations in qualities liable for controlling cholesterol levels can prompt familial hypercholesterolemia, a condition related with elevated cholesterol and an expanded gamble of coronary illness.

4. **Personalized Medicine**: Understanding one's heredi-

tary profile can assist with fitting clinical mediations. Hereditary testing can distinguish explicit gamble factors, permitting medical services suppliers to foster customized anticipation and therapy plans.

5. **Lifestyle Interaction**: Hereditary qualities and way of life factors frequently collaborate. While hereditary qualities can impact your defenselessness to coronary illness, way of life decisions like eating routine, exercise, and smoking propensities can either moderate or fuel these hereditary inclinations.

6. **Risk Assessment**: Hereditary testing can give bits of knowledge into a singular's exceptional gamble factors. This data can direct early mediations and way of life changes to lessen the gamble of coronary illness.

7. **Precision Medicine**: The area of cardiology is progressively embracing accuracy medication, which utilizes hereditary data to modify treatment procedures. Meds and treatments can be custom fitted to a patient's hereditary cosmetics for improved results.

8. **Research and Future Insights**: Continuous examination into the hereditary qualities of heart wellbeing keeps on uncovering new bits of knowledge. Researchers are recognizing more qualities related with coronary illness, which might prompt better demonstrative instruments and treatments.

9. **Preventive Measures**: Realizing your hereditary gamble variables can enable you to find proactive ways to safeguard your heart wellbeing. This could incorporate embracing a heart-solid way of life, customary check-ups, and early screenings

4

GOOD DIET PROPENSITIES:KEEPING A HEART-SOUND EATING REGIME

Keeping a heart-sound eating regimen is urgent for generally speaking cardiovascular wellbeing. Here are key standards and tips for good dieting propensities that advance heart wellbeing:

1. Pick Supplement Rich Foods:

- Focus on leafy foods, entire grains, lean proteins, and sound fats in your eating routine. These food varieties are loaded with fundamental supplements and fiber that help heart wellbeing.

2. Limit Soaked and Trans Fats:

- Diminish your admission of soaked fats tracked down in red meat, full-fat dairy items, and handled food sources. Stay away from trans fats usually found in broiled and bundled snacks as they can raise terrible cholesterol levels.

3. Decide on Solid Fats:

- Consolidate unsaturated fats, like those tracked down in olive oil, avocados, and nuts, into your eating routine. These fats can assist with bringing down terrible cholesterol and decrease the gamble of coronary illness.

4. Watch Your Sodium Intake:

- Extreme salt can raise circulatory strain, expanding the gamble of heart issues. Limit handled and pungent food sources

5. Pick Lean Proteins:

- Select lean wellsprings of protein like poultry, fish, vegetables, and tofu. Fish, especially greasy fish like salmon and trout, are wealthy in omega-3 unsaturated fats, which are astounding for heart wellbeing.

6. Control Part Sizes:

- Be aware of part sizes to abstain from gorging. Utilize more modest plates and focus on hunger signs to forestall inordinate calorie utilization.

7. Fiber-Rich Foods:

- Food varieties high in fiber, similar to entire grains, oats, beans, and natural products, can assist with bringing down cholesterol levels and manage glucose, advancing heart wellbeing.

8. Remain Hydrated:

- Drinking sufficient water is fundamental for by and large wellbeing. Pick water, natural teas, or implanted water rather than sweet beverages.

9. Limit Added Sugars:

- High sugar admission can add to corpulence and coronary illness. Limit your utilization of sweet drinks, treats, and handled snacks.

10. Adjusted Meals:

- Hold back nothing that incorporate different food sources. A balanced eating regimen gives the important supplements to help heart wellbeing.

11. Careful Eating:

- Practice careful eating by appreciating your feasts, eating gradually, and focusing on yearning and completion signs.

This can assist with forestalling indulging and further develop assimilation.*

*12. Plan and Prepare:**

- Prepare of time to go with better decisions. Cooking at home permits you to control fixings and part measure

13. Be Wary of Alcohol:

- On the off chance that you drink liquor, do as such with some restraint. Unreasonable liquor can raise pulse and add to heart issues.

14. Look for Proficient Guidance:

- On the off chance that you have explicit dietary worries or medical issue, counsel a medical care proficient or an enlisted dietitian. They can give customized counsel custom-made to your necessities.

Integrating these good dieting propensities into your way of life can altogether lessen the gamble of coronary illness and add to better generally prosperity. Recollect that consistency is critical, and little changes after some time can prompt enduring upgrades in heart wellbeing

5

PHYSICAL ACTIVITY AND HEART HEALTH: FINDING YOUR FITNESS ROUTINE

Active work is a foundation of heart wellbeing, and finding the right wellness routine can fundamentally help your cardiovascular prosperity. This is the way to find a wellness routine that works for you:

   1. Counsel Your Medical care Provider:

   - Prior to beginning any activity program, particularly assuming you have fundamental ailments, counsel your medical services supplier. They can give direction on safe activity in light of your singular requirements.

   2. Recognize Your Goals:

   - Figure out what you need to accomplish with your wellness schedule. Whether it's working on cardiovascular perseverance, shedding pounds, or lessening pressure, having clear objectives will assist you with picking the right exercises.

   3. Pick Exercises You Enjoy:

   - The best wellness routine is one that you'll stay with.

Select exercises that you really appreciate, whether it's moving, cycling, climbing, swimming, or group activities. Satisfaction makes it almost certain that you'll remain dynamic.

4. Blend Cardiovascular and Strength Training:

- A fair wellness routine ought to incorporate both cardiovascular activities (like strolling, running, or cycling) to reinforce your heart and strength preparing (utilizing loads or opposition groups) to fabricate muscle and lift digestion.

5. Begin Slowly:

- On the off chance that you're new to practice or getting once again into it after a break, start with low-force exercises. Progressively increment the length and force over the long run to keep away from injury.

6. Set a Schedule:

- Consistency is vital. Lay out a normal exercise plan that squeezes into your everyday daily practice. Go for the gold 150 minutes of moderate-power high-impact action each week.

7. Blend It Up:

- Assortment forestalls weariness as well as difficulties different muscle gatherings. Attempt various exercises to keep your wellness routine intriguing.

8. Plan and Get ready Heart-Sound Meals:

- Plan your dinners and snacks somewhat early, making it more straightforward to pick nutritious choices over inexpensive food or handled snacks.

9. Take part in Ordinary Actual Activity:

- Integrate ordinary activity into your daily practice. Go for the gold 150 minutes of moderate-power oxygen consuming movement or 75 minutes of lively force high-impact action every week, alongside muscle-reinforcing exercises.

10. Pick Exercises You Enjoy:

- Select proactive tasks that you see as agreeable and reasonable, like strolling, moving, cycling, or swimming.

11. Get Adequate Sleep:

- Focus on quality rest, holding back nothing hours out of every evening. Unfortunate rest can adversely influence digestion and heart wellbeing.

12. Oversee Pressure Effectively:

- Persistent pressure can add to unfortunate dietary patterns. Practice pressure decrease procedures like reflection, yoga, or profound breathing activities.

13. Screen Your Progress:

- Keep a diary or utilize a versatile application to follow your feasts, exercise, and weight changes. Normal self-observing can assist you with remaining focused.

14. Look for Support:

- Share your heart weight objectives with companions, family, or a medical services proficient who can give direction, consolation, and responsibility.

15. Be Patient and Persistent:

- Practical weight the board takes time. Anticipate mishaps however center around reliable, long haul progress toward your heart-sound weight.

16. Observe Achievements:

- Praise your triumphs en route, regardless of how little. Indulge yourself with non-food rewards like a spa day or another side interest to remain propelled.

Recall that keeping a solid heart weight is a long lasting obligation to your cardiovascular prosperity. By embracing these systems, you can uphold your heart's wellbeing, decrease the gamble of coronary illness, and partake in a superior generally speaking personal satisfaction.

6

SMOKING CESSATION:QUITTING FOR A HEALTHIER HEART

Stopping smoking is perhaps of the most significant step you can take for a better heart and by and large prosperity. Smoking is a significant gamble factor for coronary illness and numerous other medical problems. Here's the reason stopping is significant and a few hints to assist you with succeeding:

Why Stopping Smoking Matters for Heart Health:

1. **Reduced Hazard of Heart Disease:** Smoking harms veins, increments cholesterol levels, and raises circulatory strain, all of which altogether lift the gamble of coronary illness.

2. **Lowered Chance of Heart Attacks:** Smokers are two times as liable to have a coronary failure as non-smokers. Stopping decreases this gamble over the long haul.

3. **Improved Circulation:** Smoking tightens veins, diminishing blood stream and oxygen to the heart. Stopping permits

17

veins to mend and further develops course.

4.   **Decreased Hazard of Blood Clots:** Smoking makes blood bound to cluster, which can prompt perilous blockages in corridors. Stopping lessens this gamble.

5. **Lowered Hazard of Stroke:** Smoking builds the gamble of stroke, which can likewise result from compromised veins. Stopping smoking lessens the possibilities suffering a heart attack.

Ways to smoke Cessation:

1. **Set a Quit Date:** Pick a particular date to stop smoking. This can give an unmistakable objective to pursue.

2. **Seek Support:** Inform loved ones concerning your choice to stop. Their help and consolation can be priceless.

3. **Consider Nicotine Substitution Treatment (NRT):** NRT choices, similar to nicotine gum, patches, or tablets, can assist with overseeing withdrawal side effects.

4. **Prescription Medications:** Converse with your medical services supplier about doctor prescribed drugs, for example, varenicline or bupropion, which can support smoking end.

5.   **Counseling or Backing Groups:** Joining a smoking suspension program, directing, or uphold gathering can give direction and a feeling of local area.

6. **Identify Triggers:** Perceive circumstances or feelings that trigger your smoking propensity and foster better survival techniques.

7. **Stay Active:** Standard actual work can assist with decreasing desires and further develop state of mind during the stopping system.

8. **Practice Stress Management:** Learn pressure decrease procedures like profound breathing, reflection, or yoga to adapt to pressure without turning to smoking.

9. **Replace Smoking Habits:** Supplant smoking with better propensities like biting sans sugar gum, nibbling on leafy foods, or taking a walk when desires strike.

10. **Stay Persistent:** It's generally expected to encounter difficulties during the stopping system. On the off chance that you goof, don't surrender. Gain from the experience and continue to push toward your objective of a sans smoke life.

11. **Celebrate Milestones:** Recognize and remunerate yourself for arriving at sans smoke achievements. Indulge yourself with something uniquely great with the cash you've saved from not accepting cigarettes.

12. **Remember Your Why:** Remember the reasons you need to stop smoking, including further developed heart wellbeing, and use them as inspiration during testing minutes.

Stopping smoking is testing, however the advantages for your heart and by and large wellbeing are significant. By doing whatever it takes to stop and looking for help, you can essentially lessen your gamble of coronary illness and partake in a better, sans smoke life.

7

LIQUOR UTILIZATION:CONTROL AND CORONARY ILLNESS

Liquor utilization, especially with some restraint, has been a subject of interest concerning its likely consequences for coronary illness. While certain examinations recommend that moderate liquor admission might have specific cardiovascular advantages, it's critical to comprehend the subtleties and dangers related with liquor utilization for heart wellbeing:

Moderate Liquor Utilization and Heart Health:

1. **Potential Benefits:** Some examination has shown that moderate liquor utilization, particularly of red wine, might be related with a decreased gamble of coronary illness. This is frequently ascribed to intensifies like resveratrol, which might have cardioprotective properties.

2. **Improved HDL Cholesterol:** Moderate liquor admission can increment high-thickness lipoprotein (HDL) cholesterol levels, frequently alluded to as "great" cholesterol, which can

defensively affect the heart.

3. **Reduced Hazard of Blood Clots:** Liquor might have a gentle antiplatelet impact, which might actually decrease the development of blood clusters in supply routes.

Balance Is Key:

1. **Defining Moderation:** Moderate liquor utilization is regularly characterized as dependent upon one beverage each day for ladies and up to two beverages each day for men. A standard beverage in the US contains around 14 grams of unadulterated liquor.
   6. Lose Abundance Weight:**
   - Shedding overabundance weight can decidedly affect both LDL and HDL cholesterol levels. Indeed, even a humble weight reduction can have an effect.

7. Limit Liquor Intake:
   - Assuming you drink liquor, do as such with some restraint. Unnecessary liquor can raise fatty substance levels and affect heart wellbeing.

8. Stop Smoking:
   - Smoking brings down HDL cholesterol and harms veins, making it a significant gamble factor for coronary illness. Stopping smoking is fundamental for further developing cholesterol levels and generally speaking heart wellbeing.

9. Medications:
   - In the event that way of life changes aren't adequate,

your medical services supplier might recommend cholesterol-bringing down drugs like statins. Accept these drugs as coordinated and go to normal subsequent arrangements.

10. Oversee Stress:
   - Ongoing pressure can influence cholesterol levels. Utilize pressure decrease procedures like contemplation, yoga, or profound breathing activities to actually oversee pressure.

11. Remain Hydrated:
   - Drinking a lot of water upholds by and large wellbeing, including cardiovascular wellbeing.

12. Customary Check-Ups:
   - Plan customary check-ups with your medical care supplier to screen your cholesterol levels and generally heart wellbeing. This is particularly significant on the off chance that you have a family background of coronary illness or related conditions.

13. Limit Trans Fats:
   - Trans fats are tracked down in many handled and broiled food varieties. Stay away from these whenever the situation allows, as they can raise LDL cholesterol levels.

By following these procedures and settling on heart-sound decisions, you can bring down LDL cholesterol and raise HDL cholesterol levels, lessening your gamble of coronary illness and advancing long haul cardiovascular prosperity. Continuously talk with your medical care supplier for customized direction and proposals in light of your singular wellbeing profile.

8

MAINTAING A HEALTHY WEIGHT:STATEGIES FOR SUCCESS

Keeping a solid heart weight is crucial for cardiovascular wellbeing and generally speaking wellbeing. Here are a few powerful procedures to help you accomplish and support a weight that upholds your heart's prosperity:

1. Grasp Your Sound Weight Range:

- Talk with a medical care proficient to decide a solid weight territory for your age, level, and body type. This gives a reasonable objective to go for the gold.

2. Set Reasonable Goals:

- Lay out feasible, gradual weight reduction or upkeep objectives. Little, feasible changes are bound to prompt achievement.

3. Focus on Heart-Sound Foods:

- Center around a heart-sound eating routine wealthy in organic products, vegetables, entire grains, lean proteins (like poultry, fish, beans, and tofu), and unsaturated fats (like olive oil, avocados, and nuts). Lessen your admission of immersed and trans fats.

4. Control Piece Sizes:

- Focus on segment sizes to abstain from gorging. Utilizing more modest plates and utensils can assist you with overseeing segments successfully.

5. Limit Added Sugars and Sodium:

- Limit your utilization of food sources and refreshments high in added sugars and sodium. Inordinate sugar and salt admission can add to heart issues.

6. Remain Hydrated with Water:

- Drinking sufficient water is pivotal for in general wellbeing. It can likewise assist with controlling hunger and forestall gorging.

7. Practice Careful Eating:

- Dial back during feasts, enjoy your food, and stay away from interruptions like television or telephones. This careful methodology can assist you with perceiving when you're full and forestall overconsumption.

8. Plan and Get ready Heart-Sound Meals:

- Plan your dinners and snacks somewhat early, making it simpler to pick nutritious choices over inexpensive food or handled snacks.

9. Take part in Normal Actual Activity:

- Integrate normal activity into your daily schedule. Hold back nothing 150 minutes of moderate-force oxygen consuming movement or 75 minutes of fiery power high-impact action every week, alongside muscle-reinforcing exercises.

10. Pick Exercises You Enjoy:

- Pick proactive tasks that you see as pleasant and manageable, like strolling, moving, cycling, or swimming.

11. Get Adequate Sleep:

- Focus on quality rest, holding back nothing hours out of every evening. Unfortunate rest can adversely influence digestion and heart wellbeing.

12. Oversee Pressure Effectively:

- Ongoing pressure can add to undesirable dietary patterns. Practice pressure decrease methods like contemplation, yoga, or profound breathing activities.

13. Screen Your Progress:

- Keep a diary or utilize a versatile application to follow your dinners, exercise, and weight changes. Ordinary self-observing can assist you with remaining focused.

14. Look for Support:

- Share your heart weight objectives with companions, family, or a medical services proficient who can give direction, consolation, and responsibility.

15. Be Patient and Persistent:

- Feasible weight the board takes time. Anticipate mishaps however center around reliable, long haul progress toward your heart-sound weight.

16. Observe Achievements:

- Praise your victories en route, regardless of how little. Indulge yourself with non-food rewards like a spa day or another side interest to remain persuaded.

Recollect that keeping a sound heart weight is a long lasting obligation to your cardiovascular prosperity. By taking on these techniques, you can uphold your heart's wellbeing, decrease the gamble of coronary illness, and partake in a superior generally personal satisfaction

9

STRESS MANAGEMENT:REDUCING IT'S IMPACT ON THE HEART

1. Grasping the Association:

Stress sets off the body's "survival" reaction, causing an expansion in pulse and circulatory strain. After some time, these physiological changes can negatively affect your heart and increment the gamble of cardiovascular illnesses, including hypertension and respiratory failures.

2. Distinguish Stressors:

The most vital phase in overseeing pressure is distinguishing its sources in your day to day existence. These can be business related, individual, or even monetary. When you pinpoint the stressors, you can find designated ways to address them.

3. Practice Care and Unwinding:

Care methods, like contemplation and profound breathing activities, can assist with quieting your psyche and lessen pressure. Ordinary practice can bring down your pulse and circulatory strain, advancing heart wellbeing.

4. Remain Dynamic:

Practice is a strong pressure minimizer. Participating in actual work discharges endorphins, which are regular temperament lifters. It likewise reinforces your cardiovascular framework, making your heart stronger to stretch.

5. Keep a Sound Eating regimen:

Eating a decent eating regimen wealthy in organic products, vegetables, entire grains, and incline proteins can help your heart. Stay away from unnecessary utilization of handled food sources, sweet tidbits, and caffeine, as they can compound pressure.

6. Focus on Rest:

Sufficient rest is essential for stress the executives and heart wellbeing. Go for the gold long stretches of value rest each night to guarantee your body can recuperate and re-energize.

7. Social Help:

Try not to underrate the force of social associations. Investing energy with companions and friends and family, discussing your thoughts, and looking for help can assist with diminishing feelings of anxiety.

8. Using time productively:

Powerful using time effectively can decrease the sensation of being overpowered. Coordinate your errands, put forth boundaries, and designate time for unwinding and taking care of oneself.

9. Look for Proficient Assistance:

In the event that pressure is seriously influencing your life and wellbeing, make sure to a medical care proficient or specialist. They can give direction, treatment, or drug when important.

10. Remain Informed:

Remain informed about the most recent exploration on pressure and heart wellbeing. Understanding the science behind the association can rouse you to make positive way of life changes.

Stress can significantly affect your heart, however you have the ability to decrease its impact through way of life changes and stress the executives procedures. By distinguishing stressors, rehearsing care, keeping a sound way of life, and looking for help when required, you can safeguard your heart and have a more joyful, better existence. Keep in mind, your heart merits the consideration and consideration it requirements to flourish.

10

BLOOD PRESSURE MANAGEMENT: KEEPING IT IN CHECK

Keeping up with sound pulse is vital for in general prosperity. Hypertension, or hypertension, is a quiet however possibly perilous condition that can prompt serious medical problems. Luckily, there are powerful techniques for overseeing and controlling pulse. In this article, we'll investigate the significance of circulatory strain the board and give commonsense tips to holding it within proper limits.

Understanding Circulatory strain:

Pulse is the power of blood against the walls of your courses as your heart siphons it around your body. It's deliberate in millimeters of mercury (mm Hg) and comprises of two numbers: systolic (the top number) and diastolic (the base number). Ordinary circulatory strain is commonly around 120/80 mm Hg.

The Risks of Hypertension:

Hypertension can harm your veins, heart, cerebrum, and

other indispensable organs. Over the long run, it expands the gamble of coronary illness, stroke, kidney issues, and that's just the beginning. The issue is that hypertension frequently slips through the cracks since it seldom causes recognizable side effects. Ordinary circulatory strain observing is fundamental for early identification.

Tips for Pulse The board:

1. **Healthy Diet:** Consume an eating regimen wealthy in natural products, vegetables, entire grains, lean protein, and low-fat dairy. Lessen sodium (salt) consumption, as overabundance salt can raise circulatory strain.

2. **Regular Exercise:** Hold back nothing 150 minutes of moderate high-impact action or 75 minutes of lively movement each week. Practice assists lower with blooding pressure and works on by and large cardiovascular wellbeing.

3. **Maintain a Solid Weight:** Losing even a couple of pounds can essentially affect pulse. Go for the gold inside the sound reach.

4. **Limit Alcohol:** Extreme liquor utilization can raise circulatory strain. Assuming you drink, do as such with some restraint.

5. **Quit Smoking:** Smoking harms veins and can add to hypertension. Look for help to stop if necessary.

6. **Stress Management:** Constant pressure can raise circulatory strain. Practice unwinding strategies like profound

breathing, reflection, or yoga.

7. **Regular Check-ups:** Visit your medical care supplier for normal check-ups and pulse estimations. Heed their guidance taking drugs whenever recommended.

8. **Monitor at Home:** Consider a home circulatory strain screen to follow your readings between specialist's visits. Share these with your medical services supplier.

9. **Medication:** In the event that way of life changes aren't sufficient, your primary care physician might endorse drug to bring down pulse. Accept it as coordinated.

Circulatory strain the board is indispensable for a sound life. By taking on a heart-solid way of life and observing your pulse routinely, you can essentially decrease your gamble of hypertension-related intricacies. Keep in mind, little changes can have a major effect in holding your pulse under control and protecting your drawn out wellbeing.

11

CHOLESTEROL CONTROL:BRINGING DOWN LDL AND RAISING HDL

Cholesterol is a crucial substance in our bodies, however lopsided characteristics in its levels can prompt medical conditions. Two kinds of cholesterol are frequently talked about: LDL (low-thickness lipoprotein) and HDL (high-thickness lipoprotein). LDL is thought of "awful" cholesterol since significant levels can expand the gamble of coronary illness, while HDL is known as "great" cholesterol since it helps eliminate overabundance cholesterol from the circulatory system. Here are a few techniques to control cholesterol by bringing down LDL and raising HDL:

1. **Dietary Choices:**
   - **Diminish Soaked Fats:** Cutoff food varieties high in immersed fats like red meat, spread, and full-fat dairy items. Decide on lean protein sources and low-fat dairy.
   - **Increment Fiber:** Food sources wealthy in solvent fiber, like oats, beans, and natural products, can assist with bringing down LDL cholesterol.

- **Sound Fats:** Consolidate unsaturated fats from sources like olive oil, avocados, and nuts, which can further develop HDL levels.

2. **Regular Exercise:**
   - Participate in somewhere around 150 minutes of moderate-power oxygen consuming activity each week. Exercise can help HDL and lower LDL cholesterol.

3. **Quit Smoking:**
   - Smoking brings down HDL levels and harms veins, making it fundamental to stop for generally heart wellbeing.

4. **Moderate Liquor Consumption:**
   - A few examinations recommend that moderate liquor consumption, particularly red wine, may raise HDL levels. Nonetheless, over the top liquor can have unfavorable wellbeing impacts, so it's ideal to talk with a medical care supplier.

5. **Weight Management:**
   - Losing abundance weight, particularly around the mid-region, can assist with further developing cholesterol levels.

6. **Medications:**
   - At times, meds like statins might be endorsed by a specialist to bring down LDL cholesterol when way of life changes are lacking.

7. **Regular Check-ups:**
   - Get customary cholesterol screenings to screen your levels and survey your gamble of coronary illness.

Recall that singular reactions to these methodologies might shift, so it's significant to talk with a medical care proficient for customized direction on cholesterol control. A comprehensive methodology, consolidating dietary changes, work out, and a sound way of life, can prompt superior cholesterol profiles and better heart

12

DIABETES MANAGEMENT AND HEART DISEASE PREVENTION

Diabetes Management:
   1. **Blood Sugar Monitoring:** Consistently screen your glucose levels as prompted by your medical services supplier. Keeping your glucose inside target ranges is vital.

2. **Healthy Diet:** Follow a reasonable eating regimen wealthy in natural products, vegetables, entire grains, lean proteins, and low-fat dairy. Limit sugar and handled food varieties.

3. **Regular Exercise:** Participate in actual work most days of the week. Go for the gold 150 minutes of moderate-power practice each week.

4. **Medications:** Accept endorsed diabetes meds as co-ordinated. Insulin, oral meds, or other injectables might be important to control glucose.

5. **Stress Management:** Stress can influence glucose levels. Practice pressure decrease strategies like reflection, yoga, or profound relaxing.

Coronary illness Prevention:
   1. **Healthy Diet:** Embrace a heart-solid eating routine low in soaked and trans fats. Incorporate food varieties like fish, nuts, entire grains, and a lot of products of the soil.

2. **Regular Exercise:** Hold back nothing 150 minutes of moderate-power high-impact practice or 75 minutes of lively activity each week. Practice keeps a sound weight and further develops heart wellbeing.

3. **Quit Smoking:** Smoking is a significant gamble factor for coronary illness. Look for help to stop smoking if necessary.

4. **Control Blood Pressure:** Hypertension is a critical gamble factor for coronary illness. Screen and deal with your pulse with drug and way of life changes if important.

5. **Manage Cholesterol:** Hold your cholesterol levels in line. A low-fat, low-cholesterol diet might be suggested, alongside drug if necessary.

6. **Regular Checkups:** Visit your medical services supplier routinely for tests and screenings to identify early indications of coronary illness or diabetes-related intricacies.

7. **Weight Management:** Accomplish and keep a solid load through diet and exercise. Abundance weight can add to both

diabetes and coronary illness.

Keep in mind, it's fundamental for work intimately with your medical services group to make a customized plan for diabetes the board and coronary illness avoidance in light of your particular necessities and clinical history

13

HEART-STRONG RECIPIES AND SUPPER ORGANIZING

Certainly! The following are a couple of heart-strong recipes and supper organizing tips to help you with keeping a sound cardiovascular structure:

Breakfast:
   1. **Oatmeal with Berries:** Cook oats with skim milk or water and top with new berries, a shower of honey, and a sprinkle of hacked nuts for added fiber and sound fats.

2. **Greek Yogurt Parfait:** Layer Greek yogurt with cut bananas, a spoonful of almond margarine, and a sprinkle of granola for a protein-squeezed breakfast.

Lunch:
   1. **Grilled Chicken Salad:** Plan grilled chicken chest, cherry tomatoes,blended greens, cucumbers, and a balsamic vinaigrette dressing for a low-fat and high-protein salad.

2. **Quinoa and Chickpea Bowl:** Join cooked quinoa, diced veggies, chickpeas, , and a tahini dressing for a fulfilling and nutritious lunch.

Dinner:

1. **Baked Salmon:** Season salmon filets with flavors, lemon juice, and a smidgen of olive oil. Get ready until flaky and present with steamed broccoli and quinoa.

2. **Vegetable Blend Fry:** Sautéed food different splendid vegetables like toll peppers, broccoli, and carrots with lean protein (tofu, chicken, or shrimp) in a light soy or teriyaki sauce.

Snacks:

1. **Mixed Nuts:** A little bundle of unsalted mixed nuts gives strong fats and protein.

2. **Hummus and Veggies:** Plunge kid carrots, cucumber cuts, and toll pepper strips into hummus for an incredible nibble.

Feast Organizing Tips:

1. **Portion Control:** Know about piece sizes to keep away from reveling. Use more unassuming plates and bowls to help with portion control.

2. **Limit Sodium:** Decline your sodium affirmation by including flavors and flavors for flavor as opposed to salt.

3. **Choose Whole Grains:** Select whole grains like natural shaded rice, quinoa, and whole wheat pasta over refined grains.

4. **Lean Protein:** Unite lean protein sources like poultry, fish, tofu, and vegetables into your dining experiences.

5. **Healthy Fats:** Consolidate wellsprings of sound fats like avocados, olive oil, and nuts in your eating routine while coordinating drenched and trans fats.

6. **Meal Prep:** Plan your blowouts and snacks early on to go with better choices speedily open.

7. **Hydration:** Stay hydrated with a great deal of water throughout the day.

Remember that a heart-strong eating routine is just a single piece of staying aware of extraordinary heart prosperity. Standard genuine work, stress the board, and doing whatever it takes not to smoke are similarly essential pieces of a heart-strong lifestyle. Persistently talk with a clinical benefits capable or an enrolled dietitian for redid dietary recommendations.

14

THE MEDITERRANEAN EATING REGIMEN:A HEART-SOLID METHODOLOGY

The Mediterranean Eating regimen is broadly perceived as a heart-solid way to deal with eating. It depends on the customary dietary examples of nations lining the Mediterranean Ocean and has been related with various medical advantages, especially for heart wellbeing. Here is an outline of the Mediterranean Eating routine:

Key Components:

1. **Abundance of Foods grown from the ground The eating routine underlines a wide assortment of brilliant products of the soil, giving fundamental nutrients, minerals, and cell reinforcements that help heart wellbeing.

2. **Healthy Fats:** It supports the utilization of sound fats, fundamentally from olive oil, which is wealthy in monounsaturated fats. Nuts, seeds, and greasy fish like salmon and mackerel are additionally wellsprings of heart-sound fats.

3. **Whole Grains:** Entire grains like entire wheat, earthy

colored rice, and oats are staples, giving fiber and supplements while assisting with directing glucose levels.

4. **Lean Proteins:** Poultry, fish, and vegetables (beans, lentils, and chickpeas) are favored wellsprings of protein, with restricted red meat utilization.

5. **Dairy:** Moderate utilization of dairy items, particularly yogurt and cheddar, gives calcium and probiotics to stomach related wellbeing.

6. **Herbs and Spices:** Mediterranean cooking depends on spices and flavors like basil, oregano, and garlic for flavor, lessening the requirement for over the top salt.

Heart-Sound Benefits:

1. **Reduced Hazard of Heart Disease:** The Mediterranean Eating routine is related with a lower hazard of coronary illness, including lower levels of LDL (terrible) cholesterol and decreased irritation.

2. **Blood Strain Control:** The accentuation on entire food sources, olive oil, and potassium-rich products of the soil can assist with bringing down pulse.

3. **Weight Management:** The eating routine's emphasis on supplement thick food varieties and part control can help with keeping a sound weight, which is fundamental for heart wellbeing.

4. **Anti-Provocative Effects:** The consideration of food sources wealthy in cell reinforcements and omega-3 unsaturated fats can decrease irritation, a gamble factor for coronary

illness.

5. **Improved Glucose Control:** Entire grains and fiber-rich food sources assist with managing glucose levels, decreasing the gamble of type 2 diabetes.

Feast Ideas:

- Barbecued Mediterranean vegetable platter with a side of hummus.
   - Heated salmon with a Mediterranean tomato and olive salsa.
   - Greek serving of mixed greens with feta cheddar, olives, and a lemon-olive oil dressing.
   - Entire wheat pasta with garlic, olive oil, and sautéed spinach.

The Mediterranean Eating routine offers a flavorful and heart-solid method for sustaining your body. It's an eating routine as well as a way of life that advances generally prosperity. Make sure to talk with a medical services proficient or dietitian prior to rolling out huge dietary improvements, particularly on the off chance that you have explicit wellbeing concerns or conditions.

15

PLANT-BASED EATING FOR HEART PROSPERITY

Plant-based eating is a sublime choice for heart prosperity as it stresses whole, plant-induced food assortments and limits or takes out animal things. This approach gives an overflow of benefits to your cardiovascular system. Here is the explanation plant-based eating is heart-strong:

1. Lower Cholesterol Levels: A plant-based diet is normally low in soaked fat, which is regularly tracked down in creature items. This can assist with lessening LDL (terrible) cholesterol levels, a huge gamble factor for coronary illness.

2. Wealthy in Fiber: Plant-based slims down are high in dietary fiber, which supports lessening cholesterol levels and keeping up with solid pulse. Fiber likewise upholds a sound weight, further helping your heart.

3. Decreased Blood Pressure: The overflow of potassium-rich food sources like products of the soil in a plant-based diet can assist with bringing down circulatory strain, diminishing the gamble of hypertension and related heart issues.

4. Mitigating Properties: Many plant food varieties are

wealthy in cell reinforcements and calming intensifies that safeguard the veins and decrease irritation, a supporter of coronary illness.

5. Weight Management: Plant-based abstains from food are frequently connected with lower calorie consumption and better body loads, which can lessen the gamble of heftiness related heart issues.

6. Further developed Glucose Control: Plant-based consumes less calories are normally low in refined sugars and refined carbs, making them compelling at directing glucose levels and diminishing the gamble of diabetes, which is a coronary illness risk factor.

7. Solid Fats: While plant-based eats less carbs limit immersed fats, they integrate sound fats from sources like avocados, nuts, seeds, and olive oil, which support heart wellbeing.

8. Diminished Hazard of Heart Disease: Studies have shown that embracing a plant-based diet can essentially decrease the gamble of coronary illness and related conditions.

Here are a few ways to take on a plant-based diet for heart wellbeing:

1. **Emphasize Foods grown from the ground Make them the underpinning of your feasts, going for the gold of varieties and types.

2. **Choose Entire Grains:** Select entire grains like quinoa, earthy colored rice, and entire wheat pasta over refined grains.

3. **Include Legumes:** Beans, lentils, and chickpeas are magnificent wellsprings of plant-based protein.

4. **Healthy Snacking:** Supplant handled snacks with entire food sources like nuts, seeds, and new natural product.

5. **Limit Handled Foods:** Limit or kill handled and sweet food varieties, as they can adversely influence heart wellbeing.

6. **Consult a Dietitian:** On the off chance that you're new to plant-based eating, consider counseling an enlisted dietitian for customized direction and feast arranging.

A very much arranged plant-based diet can give every one of the supplements your body needs while advancing heart wellbeing and generally prosperity. Continuously talk with a medical services proficient prior to rolling out critical dietary improvements, particularly in the event that you have explicit wellbeing concerns or conditions.

16

SEGMENT CONTROL: A KEY TO SMART DIETING

A Key to Smart dieting

Segment control is a pivotal part of good dieting that can assist you with keeping a decent eating regimen, control your calorie admission, and backing weight the board. Here's the reason it's fundamental and a few hints to assist you with rehearsing segment control really:

Why Piece Control Matters:

1. **Calorie Management:** Controlling piece sizes assists you with dealing with your calorie admission. Consuming a bigger number of calories than your body needs can prompt weight gain and related medical problems.

2. **Balanced Nutrition:** Legitimate piece control guarantees you get a reasonable blend of supplements. It permits you to remember different food varieties for your eating regimen, which is fundamental for generally speaking wellbeing.

3. **Prevents Overeating:** Curiously large parcels can

prompt gorging, regardless of whether you're eating quality food sources. Segment control assists you with perceiving when you're full and forestall inordinate utilization.

Ways to rehearse Part Control:

1. **Use More modest Plates:** Utilizing more modest plates can fool your brain into believing you're eating more significant parts, assisting with segment control.

2. **Read Sustenance Labels:** Focus on serving sizes on nourishment names to try not to inadvertently consume bigger bits than suggested.

3. **Measure Your Food:** Use estimating cups, a food scale, or regular items (e.g., a tennis ball for a part of pasta) to check serving sizes precisely.

4. **Divide Your Plate:** Picture your plate partitioned into segments. Fill half with vegetables, one-quarter with lean protein, and one-quarter with entire grains or bland food varieties.

5. **Control Snacking:** Part out snacks into little holders or sacks to try not to thoughtlessly eat from bigger bundles.

6. **Share Eatery Meals:** While feasting out, split dishes with a companion or request a to-go compartment to save a piece before you begin eating.

7. **Listen to Your Body:** Focus on yearning and completion prompts. Quit eating when you're fulfilled, not when the plate is unfilled.

8. **Plan Ahead:** Plan your feasts and snacks ahead of time, so you're less inclined to gorge when you're ravenous and in a rush.

9. **Stay Hydrated:** Some of the time thirst is confused with hunger. Hydrate previously and during dinners to assist

with controlling your craving.

10. **Practice Careful Eating:** Delayed down and relish each nibble. This permits you to partake in your food completely and perceive when you're fulfilled.

Recollect that piece control doesn't mean denying yourself. About finding the right equilibrium upholds your wellbeing and health objectives. By rehearsing segment control, you can partake in a wide assortment of food sources while keeping a solid and feasible eating design

17

PERUSING FOOD MARKS:SETTLING ON INFORMED DECISIONS

Perusing food names is an important expertise for settling on informed decisions about the food varieties you devour. Food marks give fundamental data about the healthful substance, fixings, and serving sizes of items. This is an aide while heading to peruse food names really:

1. Serving Size: Start by taking a gander at the serving size recorded at the highest point of the name. It lets you know how much food that the sustenance realities depend on. Know about the serving size, as it can change starting with one item then onto the next and may not mirror the sum you regularly eat.

2. Calories: Check the quantity of calories per serving. This assists you with understanding the energy content of the food and how it squeezes into your everyday calorie admission.

3. Supplements to Limit:
   - **Immersed and Trans Fat:** Cutoff your admission of

soaked and trans fats, as they can raise cholesterol levels and increment the gamble of coronary illness.

   - **Sodium:** Watch out for high sodium levels, as unnecessary salt admission can prompt hypertension.

   - **Added Sugars:** Search for added sugars in the fixing list. Restricting added sugars is significant for generally speaking wellbeing.

4. Supplements to Maximize:

   - **Dietary Fiber:** Hold back nothing in dietary fiber, as it upholds absorption and assists you with feeling full.

   - **Protein:** Search for wellsprings of fit protein, which is significant for muscle wellbeing and satiety.

   - **Nutrients and Minerals:** Check for the presence of fundamental nutrients and minerals like vitamin D, calcium, iron, and potassium.

5. % Everyday Worth (%DV): The %DV demonstrates how much a supplement in one serving of the food adds to your day to day consumption in light of a 2,000-calorie diet. It can assist you with deciding whether a food is high or low in a specific supplement. Go for the gold higher %DV for fundamental supplements like fiber, nutrients, and minerals and lower %DV for soaked fat, trans fat, and sodium.

6. Fixing List: The fixing list shows every one of the parts in the item, with the most plentiful fixing recorded first. Look out for added sugars, undesirable fats, and fake added substances. Food sources with more limited fixing records and effectively conspicuous fixings are in many cases better decisions.

7. Allergens: Food names regularly feature normal allergens like nuts, soy, dairy, and wheat, making it simpler for people with food sensitivities or aversions to distinguish possible dangers.

8. Wellbeing Claims: Be wary of wellbeing claims on bundling, as they can in some cases be deluding. Center around the sustenance realities and fixing list for exact data.

By perusing food marks cautiously, you can pursue informed decisions that line up with your dietary objectives and in general wellbeing. It's a fundamental expertise for advancing a reasonable and nutritious eating regimen.

18

NORMAL WELLBEING TESTS: OBSERVING YOUR HEART WELLBEING

Normal wellbeing tests are fundamental for observing your heart wellbeing and keeping up with generally prosperity. Here's the reason they matter:

1. **Early Detection:** Routine exams can distinguish risk factors and early indications of coronary illness, for example, hypertension or cholesterol levels, before they lead to difficult issues.

2. **Preventive Care:** Specialists can give direction on way of life changes, like eating regimen and exercise, to bring down your gamble of coronary illness and keep your heart sound.

3. **Medication Management:** Assuming that you're now taking meds for heart conditions, tests guarantee your remedies are working successfully and your doses are suitable.

4. **Screening Tests:** Customary exams might incorporate tests like EKGs or stress tests to evaluate your heart's capability and recognize abnormalities.

5. **Blood Tension Monitoring:** Hypertension is a significant gamble factor for coronary illness. Ordinary tests take into consideration steady checking and early mediation.

6. **Cholesterol Levels:** Following your cholesterol levels can assist with forestalling plaque development in your supply routes, diminishing the gamble of coronary failures and strokes.

7. **Diabetes Management:** For those with diabetes, tests assist with overseeing glucose levels, as uncontrolled diabetes can add to heart issues.

8. **Weight Management:** Keeping a solid weight is urgent for heart wellbeing. Customary tests can offer direction on weight the executives procedures.

9. **Smoking Cessation:** In the event that you smoke, your PCP can offer help and assets to stop, as smoking is a critical gamble factor for coronary illness.

10. **Stress Management:** Persistent pressure can influence heart wellbeing. Talking about pressure the executives strategies with your medical care supplier is essential.

Keep in mind, ordinary wellbeing exams are not only for those with existing heart conditions. They are a proactive move toward forestalling coronary illness and guaranteeing your heart stays solid into the indefinite future. Talk with your medical services supplier to lay out a proper exam plan customized to your singular wellbeing needs.

19

Dietary Enhancements: What's Gainful and so forth

Dietary enhancements can be useful in specific circumstances, yet it's vital to comprehend which ones are useful and which may not give huge advantages. Here is a breakdown:

Helpful Dietary Supplements:

1. **Multivitamins:** These can assist with filling supplement holes in your eating routine, particularly assuming you have explicit dietary limitations or lacks.

2. **Vitamin D:** Many individuals have inadequate vitamin D levels, and enhancements can assist with keeping up with bone wellbeing, support the invulnerable framework, and possibly lessen the gamble of constant sicknesses.

3. **Omega-3 Greasy Acids:** Fish oil supplements, wealthy in omega-3s, may assist with bringing down fatty substances, diminish irritation, and backing heart and cerebrum wellbeing.

4. **Calcium:** Helpful for those with a lack of calcium or those in danger of osteoporosis, however it's not unexpected better to get calcium from dietary sources whenever the situation allows.

5. **Iron:** Iron enhancements are fundamental for people with iron-inadequacy sickliness, especially ladies of childbearing age and vegans.

Possibly Advantageous in Unambiguous Situations:

1. **Probiotics:** These can support stomach wellbeing and might be advantageous for people with stomach related issues or subsequent to taking anti-microbials. Notwithstanding, their adequacy differs.

2. **Folate (Folic Acid):** Fundamental for pregnant ladies to forestall birth abandons and might be suggested for those with specific ailments.

Restricted Proof or Not Recommended:

1. **Herbal Supplements:** Numerous natural enhancements need thorough logical proof for their adequacy and can communicate with prescriptions. Counsel a medical services supplier prior to utilizing them.

2. **Weight Misfortune Supplements:** Most weight reduction supplements are inadequate or have chances. Sound eating regimen and exercise stay the best way to deal with weight the executives.

3. **Antioxidants (e.g., L-ascorbic acid, E):** While cell reinforcements are fundamental for wellbeing, enhancements may not give similar advantages as a reasonable eating routine wealthy in products of the soil.

4. **Creatine and Amino Corrosive Supplements:** These are frequently advertised to competitors for execution improvement, yet their advantages are restricted for the typical individual.

5. **Energy Supplements:** Numerous energy-supporting enhancements contain energizers that can make side impacts and are not suggested for long haul use.

Prior to taking any dietary enhancement, it's significant to:

- Talk with a medical care supplier to decide whether you have explicit inadequacies or ailments that warrant supplementation.
   - Pick legitimate brands and items that have been tried for quality and security.
   - Stay away from uber dosing, as exorbitant admission of specific nutrients and minerals can make unfriendly impacts.
   - Recall that enhancements ought to supplement a fair eating routine, not supplant it.

Eventually, a balanced and various eating routine remaining parts the establishment for good wellbeing, and enhancements ought to be utilized shrewdly and under proficient direction when essential.

20

Medications for Heart Disease Prevention

Drugs assume a critical part in coronary illness counteraction and the executives. Here are a few normal meds endorsed for coronary illness counteraction:

1. **Statins:** These medications lower cholesterol levels in the blood, lessening the gamble of plaque development in the veins. They are frequently recommended to people with elevated cholesterol or those in danger of coronary illness.

2. **Aspirin:** Low-portion anti-inflamatory medicine can assist with forestalling blood clusters, which can prompt coronary failures and strokes. It's frequently suggested for people with a background marked by coronary illness or certain gamble factors.

3. **Blood Tension Medications:** Different classes of prescriptions, including ACE inhibitors, beta-blockers, diuretics, and calcium channel blockers, are utilized to oversee hypertension.

Controlling circulatory strain is crucial for heart wellbeing.

4. **Antiplatelet Agents:** Other than anti-inflamatory medicine, drugs like clopidogrel (Plavix) are recommended to forestall blood clumps and decrease the gamble of coronary failures and strokes.

5. **Beta-Blockers:** These prescriptions lower circulatory strain and diminish the heart's responsibility. They are much of the time utilized after a coronary failure and can likewise assist with overseeing conditions like angina and arrhythmias.

6. **ACE Inhibitors and ARBs:** These medications are utilized to treat hypertension and cardiovascular breakdown. They can assist with loosening up veins and further develop heart capability.

7. **Nitrates:** Nitrates, for example, dynamite, assist with widening veins, expanding blood stream to the heart. They are utilized to ease chest torment (angina).

8. **Antiarrhythmics:** These medications are endorsed to oversee sporadic heart rhythms (arrhythmias) and can assist with forestalling risky heart rhythms.

9. **Anticoagulants:** Meds like warfarin or more up to date anticoagulants (e.g., rivaroxaban) are recommended to forestall blood clusters, particularly in people with conditions like atrial fibrillation.

10. **Cholesterol Retention Inhibitors:** Prescriptions like

ezetimibe (Zetia) can be endorsed close by statins to additional lower cholesterol levels.

It's vital to take note of that the decision of drug relies upon a singular's particular gamble variables and clinical history. These drugs are much of the time utilized in mix with way of life changes, like a heart-solid eating routine, standard activity, and smoking discontinuance, to accomplish the best outcomes in coronary illness counteraction and the board. Continuously talk with a medical care supplier for customized direction taking drugs choices and doses.

21

Cardioprotective Supplements: A More critical Look

Cardioprotective supplements are a gathering of nutrients, minerals, and cell reinforcements that assume a significant part in supporting heart wellbeing and diminishing the gamble of cardiovascular sicknesses. We should investigate a portion of these fundamental supplements:

1. **Omega-3 Greasy Acids:** Found in greasy fish like salmon and pecans, omega-3 unsaturated fats have calming properties that can assist with bringing down the gamble of coronary illness. They might diminish fatty oils, lower circulatory strain, and further develop heart mood.

2. **Fiber:** Dietary fiber, tracked down in organic products, vegetables, entire grains, and vegetables, helps lower cholesterol levels, manage glucose, and keep a sound weight. It likewise adds to by and large heart wellbeing.

3. **Antioxidants (Nutrients C and E):** Cell reinforcements

safeguard the heart by lessening oxidative pressure and aggravation. L-ascorbic acid, found in citrus natural products, and vitamin E, tracked down in nuts and seeds, are instances of cancer prevention agent rich supplements.

4. **Magnesium:** This mineral assumes a part in keeping up with ordinary heart cadence and circulatory strain. It tends to be tracked down in mixed greens, nuts, and entire grains.

5. **Potassium:** An eating regimen wealthy in potassium, tracked down in bananas, yams, and beans, can assist with managing pulse and diminish the gamble of stroke.

6. **Folate (Nutrient B9):** Folate is fundamental for keeping up with sound veins and decreasing homocysteine levels, which are related with coronary illness. Mixed greens and invigorated cereals are great sources.

7. **Coenzyme Q10 (CoQ10):** This cancer prevention agent like supplement upholds energy creation in cells, including heart cells. It might assist with overseeing conditions like cardiovascular breakdown and hypertension.

8. **Garlic:** Garlic contains allicin, a compound that might be useful to bring down cholesterol levels and lessen circulatory strain, adding to heart wellbeing.

9. **Resveratrol:** Tracked down in grapes and red wine, resveratrol has been connected to further developed heart wellbeing because of its cell reinforcement and calming properties.

10. **Lycopene:** This cell reinforcement, tracked down in tomatoes and watermelon, may bring down the gamble of coronary illness by lessening LDL cholesterol levels.

Integrating these cardioprotective supplements into your eating routine through entire food varieties is a shrewd decision for heart wellbeing. A fair and differed diet that incorporates a lot of organic products, vegetables, entire grains, lean proteins, and sound fats gives the best mix of these supplements. Moreover, it's fundamental to keep a sound way of life, including ordinary actual work and abstaining from smoking, to boost the advantages of these heart-defensive supplements. Continuously talk with a medical services supplier or nutritionist for customized dietary proposals in light of your particular wellbeing needs and objectives

<h1 style="text-align:center">22</h1>

Understanding Heart Medications: Types and Usage

Heart meds assume a significant part in overseeing different cardiovascular circumstances, assisting patients with keeping up with heart wellbeing and work on their personal satisfaction. These prescriptions are recommended by medical care experts in light of a singular's particular condition and clinical history. Here is an outline of normal kinds of heart drugs and their utilization:

1. **Beta-Blockers**: Beta-blockers, like metoprolol and atenolol, lessen pulse and circulatory strain. They are ordinarily used to treat hypertension, angina, and heart musicality issues. By diminishing the responsibility on the heart, they can assist with further developing heart capability and lessen the gamble of coronary episodes.

2. **ACE Inhibitors (Angiotensin-Changing over Protein Inhibitors)**: ACE inhibitors like enalapril and lisinopril are utilized to bring down pulse and diminish stress on the heart.

They are likewise recommended for cardiovascular breakdown and may further develop heart capability over the long run.

3. **ARBs (Angiotensin II Receptor Blockers)**: Like ACE inhibitors, ARBs like losartan and valsartan assist with bringing down circulatory strain and can be utilized to treat cardiovascular breakdown. They work by obstructing the impacts of a chemical that river veins.

4. **Diuretics**: Diuretics, including furosemide and hydrochlorothiazide, assist with eliminating overabundance salt and liquid from the body. They are frequently used to oversee conditions like congestive cardiovascular breakdown and hypertension.

5. **Calcium Channel Blockers**: These meds, as amlodipine and verapamil, loosen up veins and lessen the heart's responsibility. They are recommended to treat hypertension, angina, and certain arrhythmias.

6. **Antiplatelet Agents**: Meds like headache medicine and clopidogrel forestall blood clumps from framing. They are fundamental for people in danger of coronary episodes or strokes.

7. **Anticoagulants**: Anticoagulants like warfarin or more current specialists like dabigatran assist forestall blood clusters in people with atrial fibrillation or different circumstances that increment the gamble of clump arrangement.

8. **Cholesterol-Bringing down Medications**: Statins like

atorvastatin and rosuvastatin are utilized to bring down cholesterol levels, diminishing the gamble of atherosclerosis and coronary illness.

9. **Nitrates**: Nitrates, like dynamite, are vasodilators that extend veins. They assist with alleviating angina side effects by expanding blood stream to the heart.

10. **Digitalis**: Digoxin is a medicine that reinforces the heart's constrictions. It is basically utilized for cardiovascular breakdown and certain arrhythmias.

Understanding the appropriate use of these prescriptions is urgent. Patients ought to adhere to their medical care supplier's directions cautiously, accept meds as endorsed, and go to normal check-ups. Moreover, way of life changes like a heart-sound eating regimen, customary activity, and stress the board frequently supplement medicine treatment for better heart wellbeing.

Continuously counsel a medical services proficient for customized guidance on heart drugs and their proper utilization. Acclimations to medicine regimens ought to just be made under the direction of a clinical master to guarantee security and viability.

Cardiovascular Restoration:Post-Coronary failure Recuperation

Cardiovascular restoration is a far reaching program intended to help people in their excursion to recuperate and recover their wellbeing subsequent to encountering a respiratory failure. This complex methodology incorporates different components pointed toward working on physical, profound, and generally speaking prosperity. Here is an outline of what you can anticipate from cardiovascular restoration during post-respiratory failure recuperation:

1. **Medical Supervision**: Cardiovascular restoration starts with a careful clinical evaluation. Medical services experts, including cardiologists, attendants, and actual advisors, screen your advancement intently all through the program.

2. **Customized Exercise Regimen**: Custom-made practice plans are at the center of cardiovascular recovery. These exer-

cises steadily develop your endurance and fortitude, lessening the gamble of future heart occasions. Exercises might incorporate strolling, cycling, and strength preparing.

3. **Nutritional Guidance**: A heart-solid eating regimen is vital. Nutritionists give direction on rolling out dietary improvements that lessen cholesterol, oversee circulatory strain, and advance in general heart wellbeing.

4. **Medication Management**: Whenever endorsed, meds are firmly checked to guarantee they are viable and very much endured. Changes might be made on a case by case basis.

5. **Education and Counseling**: Training about heart wellbeing and way of life changes is a key part. Guides and care groups offer everyday encouragement and assist people with adapting to the mental effect of a coronary failure.

6. **Risk Element Assessment**: Exhaustive appraisals recognize risk factors, for example, smoking, hypertension, diabetes, and corpulence. Systems are created to moderate these dangers.

7. **Stress Management**: Methods for stress decrease are instructed to assist with dealing with close to home factors that can add to heart issues.

8. **Monitoring Progress**: Standard check-ups and tests track enhancements in heart wellbeing, giving inspiration and permitting changes in accordance with the recovery plan as the need should arise.

9. **Lifestyle Changes**: Slowly, people are urged to take on better propensities, for example, stopping smoking, keeping a sound weight, and lessening liquor utilization.

10. **Long-Term Maintenance**: Cardiovascular restoration isn't just about recuperation; it's tied in with keeping up with heart wellbeing over the long haul. The abilities and information acquired during the program are fundamental for a heart-sound life past recuperation.

11. **Family Involvement**: Backing from family and friends and family is crucial. Including them in the restoration cycle can assist with establishing a steady climate at home.

12. **Goal Setting**: Putting forth feasible objectives is a significant piece of the recovery cycle. These objectives can go from strolling a specific distance to accomplishing explicit cholesterol or pulse levels.

Cardiovascular restoration assumes a crucial part in post-respiratory failure recuperation, improving the personal satisfaction and decreasing the gamble of future heart occasions. A comprehensive methodology addresses physical, profound, and way of life parts of heart wellbeing, engaging people to assume command over their prosperity and partake in a heart-sound life

24

Stress Decrease Strategies: Yoga, Reflection, and then some

Absolutely! Stress decrease is fundamental for keeping up with mental and actual prosperity. Here are a few successful methods, including yoga and contemplation, to assist with diminishing pressure: actual prosperity. Here are a few successful methods, including yoga and contemplation, to assist with diminishing pressure:

1. **Yoga:** Yoga consolidates actual stances, breathing activities, and reflection to advance unwinding. Normal practice can further develop adaptability and decrease pressure by quieting the psyche and easing strain in the body.

2. **Meditation:** Reflection includes zeroing in your psyche on a specific item, thought, or action to accomplish mental lucidity and profound smoothness. Care contemplation, specifically, is known for lessening pressure by advancing present-second mindfulness.

3. **Deep Breathing:** Profound, slow breaths can enact the body's unwinding reaction. Attempt strategies like diaphragmatic breathing or the 4-7-8 method, where you breathe in for a count of four, hold for seven, and breathe out for eight.

4. **Progressive Muscle Relaxation:** This procedure includes straining and afterward loosening up various muscle gatherings to deliver actual pressure. It's a successful method for combatting the actual indications of stress.

5. **Mindfulness:** Integrate care into your day to day existence by focusing on the current second without judgment. It very well may be drilled while eating, strolling, or in any event, washing dishes.

6. **Aromatherapy:** Certain fragrances, similar to lavender and chamomile, have quieting impacts. Fragrant healing can be polished through medicinal balms or scented candles.

7. **Exercise:** Normal active work discharges endorphins, which are regular temperament lifters. Indeed, even a lively walk or a fast exercise can diminish pressure and work on by and large prosperity.

8. **Journaling:** Record your considerations and sentiments to acquire understanding into wellsprings of stress and foster techniques for overseeing them.

9. **Social Support:** Conversing with companions and friends and family about your stressors can give profound help. Building areas of strength for an organization is urgent for long haul

pressure decrease.

10. **Limiting Screen Time:** Unnecessary screen time, particularly via online entertainment or news sites, can add to pressure. Put down stopping points and take computerized detoxes to turn off and re-energize.

11. **Time Management:** Focus on undertakings, break them into reasonable advances, and keep away from overcommitting. Successful using time effectively can decrease the tension of approaching cutoff times.

12. **Healthy Diet:** Eating a reasonable eating routine with a lot of natural products, vegetables, and entire grains can emphatically influence your mind-set and energy levels, lessening pressure.

13. **Quality Sleep:** Hold back nothing long periods of value rest every evening. Unfortunate rest can intensify pressure, so lay out a loosening up sleep time schedule.

14. **Hobbies and Recreation Activities:** Taking part in exercises you appreciate, whether it's perusing, painting, or planting, can give a getaway from stressors and advance unwinding.

15. **Professional Help:** In the event that pressure becomes overpowering or constant, make it a point to help from an emotional wellness proficient. Treatment and directing can give significant techniques to overseeing pressure.

Recollect that finding the right blend of methods that work for you might take time, so show restraint toward yourself and focus on taking care of oneself. Coordinating these pressure decrease techniques into your day to day schedule can prompt a more joyful, better

25

Sleep and Heart Health:Sleep and Heart Health: Quality Matters Quality Matters

Rest assumes a critical part in keeping up with heart wellbeing, and the nature of your rest matters similarly as much as the amount. Here's the reason:

1. **Sleep Duration:** Go for the gold long stretches of value rest each evening. Reliably dozing close to nothing or a lot of can expand the gamble of heart issues.

2. **Sleep Apnea:** This rest problem upsets breathing during rest and is connected to hypertension and coronary illness. Treating rest apnea can further develop heart wellbeing.

3. **Deep Sleep:** Profound, helpful rest is the point at which your pulse and circulatory strain decline. It's fundamental for cardiovascular prosperity.

4. **Sleep Cycles:** Ordinary rest designs assist with keeping a sound circadian mood, which impacts heart capability and

circulatory strain guideline.

5. **Stress Reduction:** Unfortunate rest can increment stress chemicals, adding to heart issues. Unwinding procedures and better rest can assist with overseeing pressure.

6. **Weight Management:** Absence of rest can prompt weight gain, which is a gamble factor for coronary illness. Quality rest upholds a sound weight.

7. **Inflammation:** Constant unfortunate rest can set off irritation, a consider atherosclerosis and coronary illness. Great rest can diminish aggravation markers.

8. **Blood Pressure:** Sufficient rest directs pulse. Reliably unfortunate rest can prompt hypertension, a significant gamble for heart issues.

9. **Lifestyle Choices:** Individuals who rest soundly are bound to go with solid way of life decisions in regards to eat less and work out, further helping heart wellbeing.

10. **Seek Proficient Help:** On the off chance that you have rest issues or suspect rest apnea, counsel a medical care proficient. They can prescribe way of life changes or medicines to further develop both rest quality and heart wellbeing.

The nature of your rest altogether influences your heart wellbeing. Focusing on great rest cleanliness can lessen the gamble of coronary illness and advance generally prosperity.

26

Social Support: Building a Heart-Healthy Network

Social help is an essential part of keeping up with heart well-being and generally speaking prosperity. Building a heart-solid organization of loved ones can emphatically affect your cardiovascular wellbeing in more than one way:

1. **Stress Reduction:** Solid social associations offer profound help, diminishing feelings of anxiety. Lower pressure is related with a diminished gamble of coronary illness.

2. **Healthy Habits:** Being important for a strong gathering can energize sound ways of behaving like normal activity, a fair eating routine, and stopping smoking - all useful for heart wellbeing.

3. **Emotional Well-being:** Good friendly communications can support your mind-set and decrease sensations of forlornness or sorrow, which are connected to heart issues.

4. **Blood Strain Control:** Drawing in with friends and family can assist with directing pulse. Forlornness and social disengagement can prompt more severe hypertension levels.

5. **Encouragement to Look for Clinical Help:** A steady organization can rouse you to look for clinical consideration while required, prompting early location and the board of heart-related issues.

6. **Sense of Belonging:** Feeling associated with others encourages a feeling of having a place and reason, which can emphatically influence your generally speaking mental and actual wellbeing.

7. **Cardiovascular Benefits:** Studies have shown that individuals with solid social ties will quite often have better cardiovascular results and longer life expectancies.

To construct a heart-solid informal organization:

- Support existing connections.
    - Join clubs or gatherings that line up with your inclinations.
    - Volunteer or participate in local area exercises.
    - Use innovation to remain associated with friends and family, particularly in the event that distance is a hindrance.
    - Discuss transparently with loved ones about your wellbeing objectives and difficulties.
    Recollect that social help is a two-way road. Offering backing to others can likewise be useful for your own heart wellbeing by reinforcing bonds and advancing a feeling of direction inside your organization.

27

Heart-Solid Cooking Procedures

Planning heart-good feasts includes utilizing cooking methods that focus on cardiovascular prosperity. Here are some heart-solid cooking strategies to consider:

1. **Baking and Roasting:** These techniques require negligible added fats. Utilize a modest quantity of heart-solid oils or cooking splashes to forestall staying and upgrade flavor. Broiling vegetables can likewise draw out their normal pleasantness.
2. **Grilling:** Barbecuing can be a low-fat cooking strategy, particularly for lean cuts of meat and vegetables. Be wary of high-heat barbecuing to keep away from the development of possibly hurtful mixtures.
3. **Steaming:** Steaming holds the supplements in food and doesn't need added fats. It's perfect for vegetables, fish, and poultry.
4. **Poaching:** Poaching includes tenderly stewing food in fluid, frequently water or stock. It's a low-fat cooking strategy reasonable for fish and poultry.

5. **Stir-Frying:** Utilize a limited quantity of heart-solid oil and sautéed food vegetables, lean protein sources, and entire grains. The fast cooking time holds supplements.

6. **Boiling and Blanching:** Bubbling is a straightforward method for cooking grains, pasta, and vegetables. Whitening includes momentarily bubbling vegetables prior to cooling them in ice water to protect variety and supplements.

7. **Slow Cooking:** Slow cookers can make heart-quality dinners with lean meats, vegetables, and a lot of vegetables. They require negligible added fats and take into account helpful, hands-off cooking.

8. **Using Spices and Spices:** Flavor your dishes with spices and flavors rather than exorbitant salt. This diminishes sodium consumption, which is fundamental for heart wellbeing.

9. **Limiting Immersed and Trans Fats:** Pick lean cuts of meat and limit the utilization of spread, grease, and different wellsprings of undesirable fats. Pick heart-solid oils like olive, canola, or avocado oil.

10. **Portion Control:** Focus on segment sizes to abstain from indulging, which can add to weight gain and heart issues.

11. **Limiting Added Sugars:** Diminish or wipe out added sugars in recipes, particularly in treats and drinks. Consider utilizing normal sugars like honey or maple syrup with some restraint.

12. **Whole Grains:** Pick entire grains like earthy colored rice, quinoa, and entire wheat pasta rather than refined grains for added fiber and supplements.

13. **Reducing Handled Foods:** Limit handled and bundled

food varieties, which frequently contain unfortunate trans fats, high sodium levels, and added sugars.

By integrating these heart-sound preparing strategies into your feast readiness, you can make scrumptious and nutritious dishes that help cardiovascular wellbeing.

28

Liquor Free Mixed drinks and Mocktails

Liquor free mixed drinks, otherwise called mocktails, are acquiring fame because of multiple factors, including advancing dependable drinking, obliging non-consumers, and offering a reviving option in contrast to customary cocktails. Here is some happy on liquor free mixed drinks and mocktails:

1. What Are Mocktails?

Mocktails are non-cocktails intended to copy the flavors and experience of conventional mixed drinks. They are made with innovativeness and care, mixing different fixings to make invigorating flavors and surfaces.

2. Advantages of Mocktails:

- **Better Option:** Mocktails are normally lower in calories and liberated from the adverse consequences of liquor, going with them a better decision.

- **Inclusive:** They permit everybody, including non-consumers, assigned drivers, and those staying away from liquor, to partake in the social part of mixed drinks.

- **Variety:** The universe of mocktails offers vast potential outcomes, from fruity and reviving to intricate and home grown, guaranteeing there's something for everybody.

- **Hydration:** Mocktails frequently incorporate hydrating components like new squeezes, settling on them a decent decision for remaining revived.

3. Well known Mocktail Recipes:

- **Virgin Mojito:** An exemplary mix of new lime juice, mint leaves, sugar, and soft drink water, offering a lively and rejuvenating experience.

- **Pina Colada Mocktail:** Made with pineapple juice, coconut cream, and a hint of cream of coconut, giving a tropical getaway without liquor.

- **Cucumber Cooler:** New cucumber cuts, lemon juice, and soft drink water make a cool and empowering drink.

- **Berry Sparkler:** A mix of blended berry puree, shimmering water, and a sprinkle of lemon or lime juice for a fruity and bubbly treat.

4. Inventive Garnishes:

Mocktails are frequently decorated with new organic products, spices, and beautiful trimmings to improve their appearance and fragrance.

5. Facilitating Liquor Free Events:

Consider serving mocktails at your next social affair to oblige visitors with different inclinations and dietary limitations. Offer a different scope of choices to take special care of various preferences.

6. Mocktail Culture: Many bars and eateries presently have devoted mocktail menus, perceiving the interest for energizing non-alcoholic choices. This shift is adding to a more comprehensive and mindful drinking society.

7. Experimentation: Feel free to explore different avenues regarding mocktail recipes at home. Join novel flavors, spices, and flavors to make your unmistakable liquor free without concoctions.alcohol mixed drinks and mocktails are not only for nondrinkers; they give a magnificent and comprehensive method for partaking in the specialty of mixology while remaining liquor free. Whether you're facilitating a gathering, attempting to scale back liquor, or just searching for an invigorating refreshment, mocktails offer a universe of flavors and encounters to investigate

29

Heart-Solid Nibbling: Shrewd Decisions

Surely! Keeping a heart-solid eating routine includes pursuing savvy decisions, in any event, with regards to nibbling. Here are a few hints and thoughts for heart-sound eating:

1. **Choose Entire Foods**: Settle on tidbits that are as near their normal state as could really be expected. New organic products, vegetables, and entire grains are phenomenal decisions.
2. **Nuts and Seeds**: Almonds, pecans, chia seeds, and flaxseeds are wealthy in heart-solid fats, fiber, and cell reinforcements. A little modest bunch makes for a wonderful tidbit.
3. **Greek Yogurt**: Low-fat Greek yogurt is an incredible wellspring of protein and probiotics. Top it with berries or a sprinkle of honey for added character.
4. **Berries**: Blueberries, strawberries, and raspberries are loaded with cell reinforcements that can assist with lessening the gamble of coronary illness. They're additionally low in calories and high in fiber.

5. **Oatmeal**: A bowl of cereal made with entire oats is a filling nibble. It contains dissolvable fiber that can assist with bringing down cholesterol levels.
6. **Dark Chocolate**: with some restraint, dim chocolate (70% cocoa or higher) can be a heart-sound treat. It contains cancer prevention agents known as flavonoids, which might have cardiovascular advantages.
7. **Hummus and Veggies**: Plunge cut cucumbers, carrots, and chime peppers into hummus for a wonderful and nutritious bite. Hummus is produced using chickpeas, which are high in fiber and protein.
8. **Popcorn**: Air-popped popcorn is an entire grain bite that is low in calories. Skirt the margarine and select a sprinkle of wholesome yeast or your #1 spices and flavors.
9. **Avocado Toast**: Spread pounded avocado on entire grain toast and top it with cut tomatoes or a poached egg. Avocado is wealthy in monounsaturated fats, which can be great for your heart.
10. **Trail Mix**: Make your own path blend in with a blend of unsalted nuts, dried organic products, and a sprinkle of dim chocolate chips. This gives a fantastic blend of sound fats, fiber, and a bit of pleasantness.

Keep in mind, segment control is key while nibbling. Pre-segment your snacks to abstain from indulging, and attempt to adjust your decisions over the course of the day. Going with these shrewd decisions can add to a heart-sound way of life.

30

Conclusion

Wellbeing Diaries and Applications

Keeping a solid heart is a deep rooted responsibility, and monitoring your advancement is critical to progress. In this computerized age, heart wellbeing diaries and applications have become imperative apparatuses for people hoping to screen and further develop their cardiovascular prosperity. Whether you're meaning to bring down your circulatory strain, oversee cholesterol levels, or basically embrace a heart-sound way of life, these devices can have a tremendous effect in your excursion to better heart wellbeing.

The Advantages of Following Your Heart Health:

1. *Awareness and Education:* Heart wellbeing diaries and applications give important data about heart wellbeing, assisting clients with turning out to be more mindful of the variables that add to cardiovascular issues. This information enables people to settle on informed decisions and way of life changes.

2. *Consistency and Accountability:* Routinely logging your heart-related information, for example, pulse, pulse, exercise, and diet, cultivates consistency. Realizing that you're keeping tabs on your development can assist you with remaining responsible to your wellbeing objectives.

3. *Early Recognition and Prevention:* Recognizing potential issues early is vital in forestalling heart sicknesses. Numerous heart wellbeing applications offer elements like side effect following and hazard evaluation, empowering clients to distinguish advance notice signs and go to proactive lengths.

Picking the Right Heart Wellbeing Diary or App:

1. *User-Accommodating Interface:* Search for applications and diaries with an instinctive connection point that makes it simple to record and audit your information. Ease of use energizes predictable following.

2. *Data Security:* Guarantee that the application or diary you pick focuses on information security and protection. Your wellbeing data ought to be kept private and shielded from unapproved access.

3. *Customization:* Everybody's heart wellbeing venture is novel. Decide on an application or diary that permits you to put forth customized objectives and adjust to your particular necessities.

4. *Integration and Compatibility:* Some applications can adjust with wearable gadgets like wellness trackers and smartwatches, making it consistent to follow your heart wellbeing information. Check for similarity with your

current gadgets.

Top Heart Wellbeing Apps:

1. **MyFitnessPal:** This famous application offers an exhaustive stage for following eating regimen, exercise, and weight, which are urgent parts of heart wellbeing.
2. **Heart Habit:** Planned explicitly for heart wellbeing the executives, Heart Propensity assists you with checking pulse, cholesterol levels, and that's only the tip of the iceberg.
3. **Samsung Health:** Viable with Samsung gadgets, this application tracks different wellbeing measurements and gives experiences to assist you with keeping a solid heart.

Keeping tabs on your development in keeping up with heart wellbeing is a proactive move toward a more extended, better life. Heart wellbeing diaries and applications improve on the interaction as well as engage you with information and inspiration to pursue heart-solid decisions. Exploit these computerized devices, and along with a heart-sound way of life, you can shield your cardiovascular prosperity for quite a long time into the future.